ANGER MANAGEMENT FOR MEN

Strategies To Manage Emotions And

Improve Relationship

Chris Oyakhilome

TABLE OF CONTENTS

INTRODUCTION

Anger is a natural and powerful emotion that everyone experiences at some point in their lives. It can serve as a healthy response to perceived threats or injustices, motivating individuals to assert themselves and address challenging situations. However, when anger is not managed effectively, it can lead to destructive consequences for both the individual experiencing anger and those around them.

Anger management is a crucial skill, and its importance becomes even more pronounced when considering gender-specific dynamics. In the context of men, societal expectations, cultural norms, and individual experiences often contribute to unique challenges in recognizing, expressing, and managing anger.

Anger management for men involves understanding the complex interplay of biological, psychological, and social factors that contribute to the expression of anger. Men, traditionally associated with traits like strength, assertiveness, and control, may face distinct pressures in how they navigate and display their anger.

The societal narrative around masculinity sometimes discourages emotional vulnerability, framing anger as an acceptable outlet for frustration. Consequently, men may find it challenging to express anger in a healthy and constructive manner, leading to a range of negative outcomes such as strained relationships, workplace issues, and even legal troubles.

In this book 'Anger Management For Men ' Occupational Therapist Chris Oyakhilome tells What Anger Is, discuses Stages Of Anger, its Side Effects, shades light on how one can Understand And Manage Anger, delves into Self-Love Amid Anger, focuses on how one should Love Himself Enough To Forgivc Others, Let Go Grudges, gives practical example on How To Channel Anger To Something Productive, reveals template Spouses Should use in Managing Anger, x-rays Parent-Kid Anger Management, gives guides on how To Build And Maintain Healthy Relationship Void Of Conflict, stresses on The Role Of Communication In Anger Management, shares Tips On How

To Handle Difficult Situations, How To Effectively Manage Anger, says Anger has Impacts On Health, and Family, as well as giving Q&A For Support.

This comprehensive guide on anger management for men seeks to explore the various facets of anger in the male experience. It will delve into the physiological aspects of anger, the impact of societal expectations on men's emotional expression, and effective strategies for recognizing, processing, and expressing anger in a constructive way. By providing insights into the root causes of anger and offering practical tools for managing this powerful emotion, this guide aims to empower men to navigate their emotional landscapes with self-awareness and resilience. Ultimately, the goal is to foster healthier relationships, improved well-being, and a more fulfilling life for men seeking to master the art of anger management.

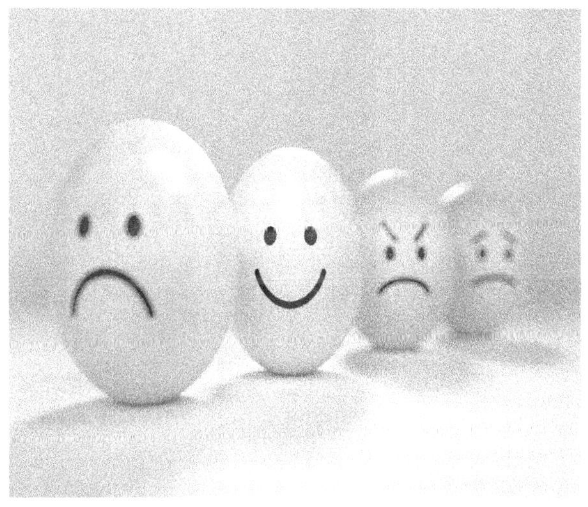

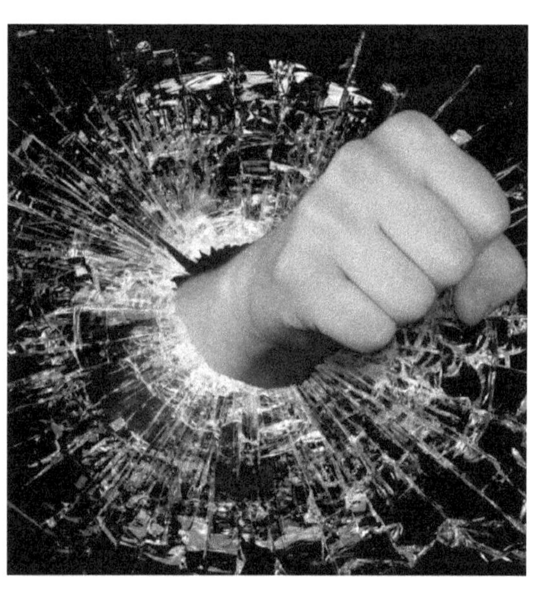

CHAPTER ONE

WHAT ANGER IS

Anger is a powerful and complex emotion that is a fundamental part of the human experience. It is a natural response to perceived threats, injustice, or frustration, and it can manifest in a variety of ways, from mild irritation to intense rage. Understanding anger, its triggers, and its consequences is crucial for emotional well-being and effective interpersonal relationships.

At its core, anger is an adaptive response that has evolved to help humans confront and overcome challenges. When faced with a threat or injustice, the body's stress response is activated, releasing hormones such as adrenaline that prepare the individual for a fight-or-flight response. This physiological reaction is often accompanied by a surge of anger, motivating the person to take action and assert themselves in the face of perceived danger.

Furthermore, while anger serves an evolutionary purpose, its expression and management can be complex. Uncontrolled or chronic anger can have detrimental effects on both physical and mental health. It has been linked to an increased risk of cardiovascular problems, weakened immune function, and mental health disorders such as depression and anxiety. Additionally, prolonged anger can strain relationships, as constant outbursts or simmering resentment creates a toxic atmosphere.

The triggers for anger vary widely and can be deeply personal. Common sources of anger include perceived injustice, frustration, disrespect, and feelings of powerlessness. Cultural and societal factors also play a role, as individuals may internalize societal norms and expectations that shape their emotional responses. Personal experiences, upbringing, and learned behaviors contribute to the development of an individual's anger management style.

The expression of anger is multifaceted and can range from assertiveness to aggression. Assertive anger involves expressing one's feelings and needs in a direct and respectful manner, while aggressive anger involves hostile and harmful actions. Passive-aggressive behavior, another manifestation of anger, involves indirect expression of hostility through sarcasm, sulking, or other subtle means. Effective anger management involves recognizing the triggers, understanding the underlying emotions, and developing healthy coping mechanisms.

One widely used approach to anger management is cognitive-behavioral therapy (CBT), which focuses on identifying and challenging distorted thought patterns that contribute to anger. By changing the way individuals perceive and interpret events, CBT helps them develop more constructive responses to anger triggers. Mindfulness and relaxation techniques, such as deep breathing and meditation, are also effective in calming the physiological arousal associated with anger.

It's essential to differentiate between healthy and unhealthy expressions of anger. While suppressing anger entirely can lead to its own set of problems, uncontrolled and aggressive outbursts can be equally harmful. Striking a balance between acknowledging and expressing anger appropriately is crucial for emotional well-being.

More so, fostering empathy and communication skills can contribute to healthier relationships and prevent conflicts that might lead to anger. Creating a supportive environment where individuals feel heard and understood can reduce the likelihood of anger escalating into destructive behavior.

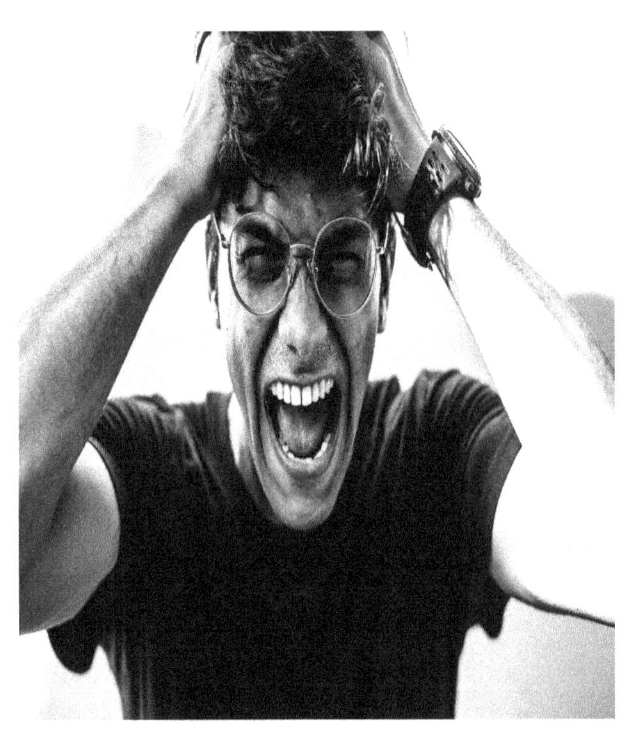

CHAPTER TWO

UNDERSTANDING AND MANAGING YOUR ANGER

Understanding and managing anger is a crucial aspect of emotional intelligence. Anger is a natural and normal human emotion, but it can become problematic when it is not effectively recognized and addressed. To understand one's anger, individuals can employ various strategies that involve self-awareness, reflection, and constructive communication.

Self-awareness is key to understanding anger. This involves recognizing the signs and triggers of anger. For instance, an individual may notice physical symptoms like a racing heart, clenched fists, or a flushed face.

By paying attention to these cues, one can start to identify patterns and understand the situations that tend to evoke anger. Keeping a journal can be a helpful tool in this process, allowing individuals to track their emotions and identify common themes.

Furthermore, understanding the underlying causes of anger is crucial. Anger is often a secondary emotion, meaning it can be a response to deeper feelings such as hurt, fear, or frustration. For example, a person who feels overlooked at work may express anger, but the root cause could be a sense of not being valued or respected. By delving into the underlying emotions, individuals can gain insights into the true source of their anger and address it more effectively.

Reflecting on past experiences of anger can also be enlightening. Identifying recurrent situations that trigger anger provides an opportunity for self-reflection. For instance, if someone consistently becomes angry during discussions about politics, it might be worthwhile to explore why those conversations are particularly challenging. Understanding the underlying beliefs and values that contribute to anger in specific situations can lead to more informed and measured responses.

More so, recognizing individual anger styles is crucial. People express anger in various ways – some may become aggressive, while others may withdraw. Understanding one's preferred style of expressing anger enables individuals to tailor their approach to managing it effectively.

For example, if someone tends to withdraw when angry, finding healthier ways to communicate their feelings without shutting down can be a constructive step. Effective communication is another essential component of understanding and managing anger. Expressing feelings assertively, without aggression, is crucial. Using "I" statements, such as "I feel frustrated when..." instead of blaming language, can promote better understanding and resolution. For instance, instead of saying, "You always ignore my ideas," one can express, "I feel unheard when my ideas are not acknowledged."

Additionally, practicing mindfulness can be beneficial. Mindfulness sometimes includes being present in the moment without judgment. Techniques such as deep breathing or meditation can help individuals stay calm in the face of anger triggers. Mindfulness allows for a pause between the stimulus and the response, providing the opportunity to choose a more thoughtful reaction.

However understanding one's anger is a multifaceted process that involves self-awareness, reflection, and effective communication. By recognizing the signs and triggers of anger, exploring underlying emotions, reflecting on past experiences, identifying individual anger styles, and practicing mindful responses, individuals can gain valuable insights into what is making them angry and develop healthier ways of managing it. This self-awareness not only fosters personal growth but also

enhances relationships and
contributes to overall emotional
well-being.

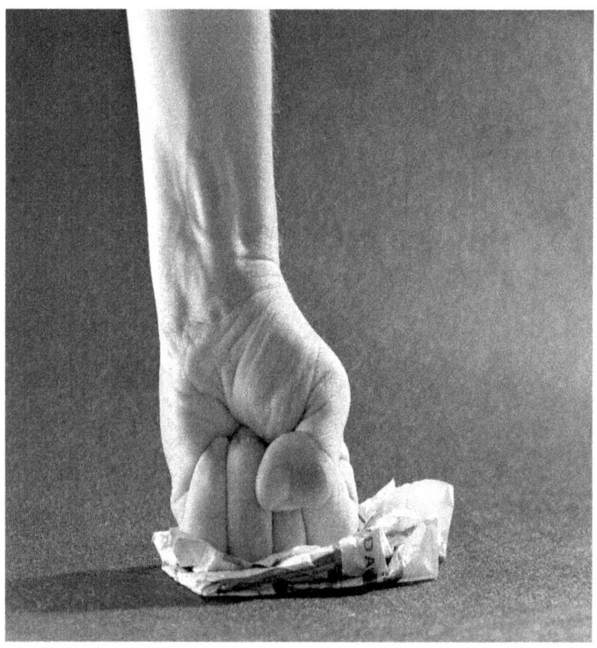

CHAPTER THREE

DYNAMICS OF ANGER

Understanding the dynamics of anger is crucial for managing and navigating through this complex emotion. Anger is a natural and universal emotion, often triggered by perceived threats, frustration, injustice, or personal offenses. It can manifest in various forms, ranging from mild irritation to intense rage. To comprehend the dynamics of anger, it's essential to explore its triggers, physiological responses, and psychological components.

Triggers:

Perceived Threats: Anger often arises in response to situations perceived as threatening, whether physically or emotionally.

Frustration: When individuals face obstacles or encounter difficulties in achieving their goals, frustration can escalate into anger.

Injustice: Perceptions of unfairness, inequality, or violations of one's rights can evoke anger.

Personal Offenses: Feeling disrespected, insulted, or harmed can trigger anger as a defense mechanism.

Physiological Responses:

Fight or Flight: Anger activates the body's "fight or flight" response, preparing it for action. This includes increased heart rate, elevated blood pressure, and the release of stress hormones like adrenaline.

Muscle Tension: Anger often leads to muscle tension, preparing the body for physical confrontation. Cognitive Changes: Anger can narrow focus, making individuals more attuned to perceived threats while impairing rational thinking. Expressive and Suppressive

Approaches:

Expressive: Some individuals express anger openly, through assertive communication or physical outlets. While this can provide a sense of release, uncontrolled expression may lead to negative consequences.

Suppressive: Others may suppress anger, avoiding confrontation or internalizing the emotion. Repressed anger can manifest in passive-aggressive behavior, impacting mental well-being.

Cognitive Components:

Cognitive Appraisal: Anger is influenced by how individuals interpret and appraise a situation. Different people may respond with anger to the same event based on their unique perspectives.

Attribution: People often attribute intentions to others, and when these intentions are perceived as negative, it can fuel anger.

Coping Mechanisms:

Adaptive Coping: Healthy anger management involves recognizing and addressing the root causes of anger, seeking solutions, and learning constructive communication.

Maladaptive Coping: Unhealthy coping mechanisms, such as aggression, passive-aggression, or substance abuse, may provide temporary relief but often exacerbate the underlying issues.

Cultural and Social Influences:

Cultural Norms: Cultural expectations and norms play a role in shaping how anger is expressed and accepted within a society.

Social Learning: Observational learning from family, peers, and society influences how individuals perceive and manage anger. Understanding the dynamics of anger enables individuals to cultivate emotional intelligence, promoting healthier responses to this powerful emotion. It involves self-awareness, empathy for others, and the development of effective coping strategies to manage and express anger constructively.

CHAPTER FOUR

CAUSES OF ANGER

Anger is a complex and multifaceted emotion that can be triggered by a variety of factors, both internal and external. Understanding the causes of anger is crucial for managing and addressing this powerful emotion. Here are some of the key factors that contribute to the emergence of anger:

Perceived Threats or Injustice:

One of the primary triggers for anger is the perception of a threat or injustice. When individuals feel that their well-being, rights, or values are being compromised, they may respond with anger as a natural defense mechanism.

Frustration:

Frustration arises when individuals encounter obstacles or challenges that impede their progress toward a goal. If these frustrations persist or accumulate, they can escalate into anger. The inability to achieve desired outcomes can be a significant source of frustration.

Unmet Needs:

When basic human needs, such as the need for love, recognition, or autonomy, are not met, it can lead to feelings of frustration and anger. People may become angry when they perceive that their fundamental needs are being ignored or neglected.

Individuals may become angry in response to perceived disrespect, humiliation, or criticism. Feeling belittled or devalued can trigger a defensive reaction in the form of anger.

Lack of Control:

A sense of powerlessness or lack of control over a situation can contribute to anger. When individuals feel that they have no influence or control over their circumstances, they may experience frustration and anger.

Past Trauma:

Previous experiences of trauma or abuse can sensitize individuals to certain triggers, making them more prone to anger when confronted with situations that remind them of past pain or injustice.

Cognitive Distortions:

Distorted thought patterns, such as overgeneralization, black-and-white thinking, or catastrophizing, can contribute to the misinterpretation of events and lead to unwarranted anger. Negative thought patterns can create a skewed perception of reality.

Biological Factors:

Biological factors, such as chemical imbalances in the brain or certain medical conditions, can influence an individual's susceptibility to anger. Hormonal changes, neurotransmitter irregularities, and genetic predispositions can all play a role.

Environmental Factors:

The environment in which an individual is raised and lives can contribute to the development of anger. Exposure to violence, social unrest, or a hostile family environment can shape how individuals express and cope with anger.

Cultural and Societal Influences:

Cultural norms and societal expectations regarding the expression of emotions can impact how individuals deal with anger. Some cultures may encourage the suppression of anger, while others may tolerate or even encourage its expression.

It's important to note that anger itself is not inherently negative; it can serve as a valuable signal that something is amiss and needs attention.

However, when anger is expressed inappropriately or becomes chronic, it can have detrimental effects on mental and physical health, relationships, and overall well-being. Learning healthy ways to manage and express anger is essential for maintaining emotional balance and fostering positive relationships.

CHAPTER FIVE

STAGES OF ANGER

Anger is a complex and universal emotion that everyone experiences at various points in life. It is a natural response to perceived threats, injustice, frustration, or violation of personal boundaries.

The process of anger unfolds in distinct stages, each contributing to the overall experience and expression of this intense emotion. Understanding these stages can be crucial for managing and mitigating the impact of anger on individuals and their relationships.

The first stage of anger is the trigger or the provocation. This initial phase involves a stimulus that is perceived as a threat or an affront to one's well-being. Triggers can vary widely, ranging from external events such as criticism or injustice to internal factors like frustration or disappointment. The interpretation of these triggers plays a vital role in determining the intensity and nature of the subsequent anger.

Following the trigger, the second stage is the arousal phase. This is characterized by the physiological and psychological responses to the perceived threat. Physiologically, the body undergoes changes such as increased heart rate, elevated blood pressure, and the release of stress hormones like cortisol.

Psychologically, there is a heightened state of alertness and a narrowing of focus on the source of the anger. This stage prepares the individual for a potential response to the perceived threat.

The third stage is the of subjective experience anger. This involves the conscious awareness of the emotion and the accompanying thoughts and feelings. Individuals may experience a range of emotions, including frustration, irritation, or even rage.

The intensity of this stage is influenced by personal and cultural factors, as well as the individual's ability to regulate and express their emotions.

The fourth stage is the expression of anger. At this point, individuals may choose to express their anger in various ways, ranging from assertive communication to aggressive behavior.

How anger is expressed can significantly impact the outcome of the situation and the relationships involved. Constructive expression involves addressing the issue at hand without causing harm, while destructive expression may lead to further conflict and damage.

The fifth stage is the aftermath or the resolution phase. This stage involves the consequences of the expressed anger and the efforts to resolve the underlying issues. If anger is managed effectively, it can serve as a catalyst for positive change, prompting individuals to address conflicts, set boundaries, or seek solutions.

However, unresolved anger can lead to lingering resentment, damaged relationships, and negative consequences for mental and physical health.

Importantly, not everyone progresses through these stages in a linear fashion. Some individuals may skip certain stages or get stuck in one, leading to chronic anger issues. Additionally, the duration of each stage can vary, with some people quickly moving through the process, while others may struggle to reach resolution.

Recognizing and managing anger effectively requires self-awareness, emotional intelligence, and coping strategies. Techniques such as deep breathing, mindfulness, and communication skills can be instrumental in navigating the stages of anger and fostering healthier responses.

Ultimately, understanding the stages of anger provides a roadmap for individuals to navigate this powerful emotion, promoting personal well-being and constructive conflict resolution.

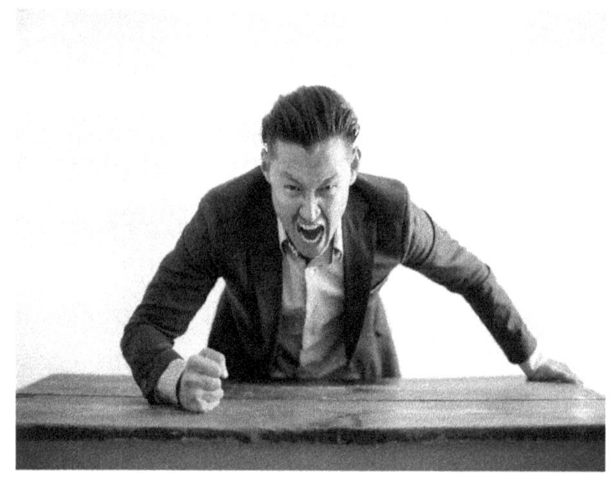

CHAPTER SIX

GENERAL EFFECTS OF ANGER

Anger is a natural and common human emotion that can arise in response to perceived threats, injustices, or frustrations. While experiencing anger is a normal part of life, it's crucial to recognize and manage it effectively, as prolonged or intense anger can have various adverse effects on both physical and mental well-being. Here is a comprehensive look at the side effects of anger:

1. Physical Health Effects:

a. Cardiovascular Issues: Intense anger can trigger the release of stress hormones, such as adrenaline, which can elevate

blood pressure and increase the
risk of heart problems.

 b. Weakened Immune System:
Chronic anger may compromise
the immune system, making
individuals more susceptible to
illnesses and infections.

c. Muscle Tension: Anger often
leads to muscle tension, which can
contribute to headaches, migraines,
and other physical discomforts.

2. Mental Health Effects:

a. Increased Stress: Anger is a
stress response that, when chronic,
can contribute to overall stress
levels and exacerbate existing
mental health conditions.

 b. Impaired Judgment: Angry
individuals may experience
impaired decision-making and may

act impulsively, leading to negative consequences.

c. Heightened Anxiety: Persistent anger can contribute to heightened anxiety levels, creating a cycle of negative emotions.

3. Interpersonal Effects:

a. Strained Relationships: Uncontrolled anger can strain relationships with family, friends, and colleagues, leading to isolation and social difficulties.

b. Communication Breakdown: Anger often hinders effective communication, making it difficult to express oneself calmly and to understand others.

c. Increased Conflict: Regular outbursts of anger can escalate conflicts, leading to a hostile environment in personal and professional settings.

4. Cognitive Effects:

a. Impaired Concentration: Anger can interfere with concentration and focus, affecting one's ability to perform tasks effectively.

b. Memory Problems: Chronic anger may contribute to memory impairment and difficulties in recalling information.

c. Negative Thought Patterns: Prolonged anger can foster negative thought patterns, making it challenging to see situations objectively and find constructive solutions.

5. Behavioral Effects:
a. Aggressive Behavior: Anger often manifests as aggression,

which can lead to verbal or physical confrontations and legal consequences.

b. Substance Abuse: Some individuals may turn to substances like alcohol or drugs to cope with anger, leading to potential addiction issues.

c. Self-Harm: In extreme cases, unmanaged anger may contribute to self-destructive behaviors, including self-harm.

6. Long-Term Consequences:

a. Chronic Health Conditions: Persistent anger has been linked to the development or exacerbation of chronic health conditions such as hypertension, heart disease, and digestive issues.

b. Mental Health Disorders:
Uncontrolled anger may contribute
to the development or worsening
of mental health disorders,
including depression and anxiety
disorders.

7. Impact on Overall Well-Being:

a. Reduced Quality of Life: The
cumulative impact of anger on
physical and mental health,
relationships, and behavior can
significantly diminish overall
quality of life.

 b. Negative Impact on
Work/Productivity: Anger can
affect professional life, leading to
decreased productivity, strained
work relationships, and potential
job loss.

8. Coping Strategies:

a. Mindfulness and Relaxation Techniques: Practices like deep breathing, meditation, and mindfulness can help manage anger.

 b. Effective Communication Skills: Learning to express feelings calmly and assertively can improve relationships and reduce conflicts.

c. Seeking Professional Help: In cases of persistent anger or difficulty in anger management, seeking the assistance of a mental health professional can be beneficial.
While anger is a normal human emotion, it is crucial to recognize its potential side effects and employ effective strategies for managing and expressing it constructively.

Developing emotional intelligence, communication skills, and coping mechanisms can contribute to a healthier and more balanced emotional life.

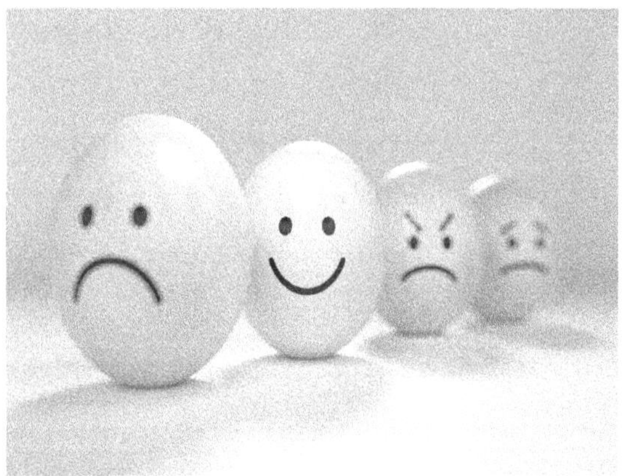

CHAPTER SEVEN

EFFECT OF ANGER ON HEALTH

Anger, when experienced frequently or intensely, can have various negative effects on a person's health. Anger management is important for several reasons, as uncontrolled or chronic anger can have significant negative effects on individuals and those around them.

It is a powerful and natural emotion that everyone experiences at some point in their lives. While it is normal to feel angry in response to certain situations, prolonged and intense anger can have significant and detrimental effects on one's health.

The link between anger and health is complex, involving both psychological and physiological factors that can impact various aspects of well-being.

One of the immediate and noticeable effects of anger on health is its impact on the cardiovascular system. When a person becomes angry, the body's stress response is activated, leading to the release of stress hormones such as adrenaline and cortisol.

These hormones cause a cascade of physiological changes, including an increase in heart rate and blood pressure. Over time, frequent episodes of anger and the associated cardiovascular changes can contribute to the development of hypertension and an increased risk of heart disease.

Chronic anger also weakens the immune system, making the body more susceptible to illnesses and infections. The prolonged release of stress hormones suppresses the immune response, reducing the body's ability to fight off viruses and bacteria. This can result in a higher incidence of illnesses and longer recovery times from common ailments.

Furthermore, the impact of anger on mental health cannot be overlooked. Persistent anger is often associated with high levels of stress and can contribute to the development or exacerbation of mental health disorders such as anxiety and depression. The constant emotional turmoil can lead to disrupted sleep patterns, fatigue, and a decreased ability to cope with daily challenges. Over time, this may contribute to the development of more serious mental health conditions.

In addition to its physiological and psychological effects, anger can also manifest in destructive behaviors that further compromise one's health. People who struggle with anger management may engage in unhealthy coping mechanisms such as substance abuse or overeating. These behaviors not only have direct negative effects on physical health but can also create a cycle of worsening anger and escalating health issues.

Relationships, both personal and professional, can suffer as a result of unchecked anger. The emotional toll of chronic anger can lead to strained relationships, social isolation, and feelings of guilt and remorse. The resulting social stress can further exacerbate the negative impact of anger on mental and physical health.

Recognizing and managing anger is crucial for mitigating its adverse effects on health. Strategies such as mindfulness, deep breathing exercises, and regular physical activity can help individuals cope with anger in a healthier way. Seeking professional support, such as therapy or counseling, can also be beneficial for those struggling to manage their anger effectively. Here are more key reasons why anger should be managed:

Increased Stress Levels: Anger triggers the body's "fight or flight" response, leading to the release of stress hormones such as cortisol and adrenaline. Prolonged exposure to these hormones can contribute to chronic stress, which is associated with a range of health problems.

Cardiovascular Issues: Intense anger can lead to a temporary increase in heart rate and blood pressure. Over time, chronic anger may contribute to the development of cardiovascular problems, such as hypertension and an increased risk of heart disease.

Weakened Immune System: Chronic anger has been linked to a weakened immune system, making individuals more susceptible to illnesses and infections.

Digestive Problems: Stress and anger can affect the digestive system, leading to issues such as indigestion, irritable bowel syndrome (IBS), and other gastrointestinal problems.

Muscle Tension and Pain: Holding onto anger can result in increased muscle tension, leading to headaches, migraines, and other physical discomforts. Chronic muscle tension can contribute to conditions like tension-type headaches and musculoskeletal pain.

Sleep Disturbances: Anger and stress can interfere with sleep patterns, leading to difficulties falling asleep or staying asleep. Poor sleep quality, in turn, can have a negative impact on overall health.

Social Consequences: Frequent anger and aggressive behavior can strain relationships with family, friends, and colleagues. This social isolation or strained relationships can contribute to stress and negatively impact mental health.

Increased Risk-Taking Behaviors:
Some individuals may engage in
risky behaviors as a way of coping
with anger, such as substance
abuse or aggressive actions, which
can further jeopardize their health.

Relationships:

Interpersonal Relationships:
Uncontrolled anger can strain
relationships with family, friends,
and colleagues. It may lead to
conflicts, damaged trust, and a
breakdown in communication.
Learning to manage anger can
foster healthier and more positive
relationships.

Workplace Success:

Professional Consequences: In a
work environment, unmanaged

anger can negatively impact career progression and job satisfaction. It may lead to conflicts with colleagues, superiors, or clients, potentially jeopardizing one's professional reputation and opportunities.

Emotional Well-being:

Mental Health: Uncontrolled anger is often linked to mental health issues such as anxiety and depression. Managing anger contributes to better emotional well-being and overall mental health.

Legal Consequences:

Legal Issues: Expressing anger inappropriately may lead to legal consequences, such as assault or property damage. Learning to manage anger can help individuals avoid legal troubles and maintain a law-abiding lifestyle.

Personal Growth:

Self-Improvement: Anger management is a crucial aspect of personal development. Learning to understand, express, and cope with anger in a constructive way contributes to self-awareness and emotional intelligence.

Improved Decision-Making:

Clarity of Thought: Anger can cloud judgment and impair decision-making abilities. Managing anger allows individuals to think more clearly and make better-informed choices in various aspects of life.

Enhanced Communication:

Effective Communication: Anger often leads to poor communication. Learning to manage anger helps individuals express themselves more clearly and assertively without resorting to aggressive or hostile behavior.

Conflict Resolution:

Resolving Conflicts: Anger can escalate conflicts, making resolution more challenging. Effective anger management techniques can facilitate conflict resolution and promote understanding between parties.

Positive Role Modeling:

Influence on Others:
Demonstrating effective anger management sets a positive example for others, especially for children and younger individuals who may learn from adult behavior.Top of Form
Managing anger is essential for maintaining physical and mental health, fostering positive relationships, succeeding in the workplace, and contributing to personal growth and well-being. It involves developing coping strategies, communication skills, and emotional regulation techniques to navigate challenges in a constructive manner.

The relationship between anger and health is multifaceted and extends beyond the immediate emotional experience. Chronic anger has the potential to negatively impact cardiovascular health, weaken the immune system, and contribute to the development of mental health disorders.

Destructive behaviors associated with anger can further compromise overall well-being. Recognizing the signs of anger, implementing effective coping strategies, and seeking support when needed are crucial steps in maintaining both mental and physical health in the face of this powerful emotion.
It's important to note that not all anger is harmful. It's a normal and often healthy emotion when expressed constructively.
However, chronic or intense anger that is not managed effectively can contribute to various health issues. Seeking support from mental health professionals, practicing

stress management techniques, and
developing healthy coping
mechanisms are essential for
maintaining overall well-being.

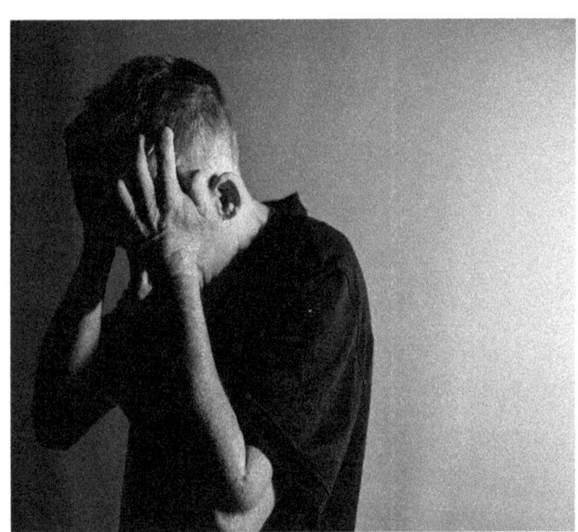

CHAPTER EIGHT

EFFECT OF ANGER ON FAMILY

Anger is a powerful and complex emotion that can have profound effects on individuals and their relationships, including within families. When not managed effectively, anger can lead to a range of negative consequences for family dynamics. Here are several ways in which anger can impact a family:

Communication Breakdown:

Anger often disrupts effective communication within a family. When individuals are angry, they may express themselves in hurtful or aggressive ways, making it difficult for others to understand their perspective. This breakdown in communication can sometimes lead to misunderstandings, resentment, and a lack of emotional connection which is not healthy for any family.

Conflict and Hostility:

Unresolved anger can escalate into frequent conflicts and increased hostility within the family. Continuous arguments and tension can create a toxic environment, making it challenging for family members to feel safe and supported at home.

Emotional Distance:

Chronic anger can create emotional distance between family members. The fear of encountering anger may lead individuals to withdraw emotionally, avoiding open and honest communication. This emotional distance can erode the sense of unity and closeness that is crucial for a healthy family dynamic.

Impact on Children:

Children are particularly vulnerable to the effects of anger within the family. Witnessing frequent displays of anger or experiencing anger directed at them can have lasting emotional and psychological consequences. It may lead to feelings of insecurity, anxiety, and a distorted understanding of healthy relationships.

Health Consequences:

The stress associated with ongoing anger within a family can have negative health effects on all members. Chronic stress has been linked to various physical and mental health issues, including cardiovascular problems, weakened immune systems, and anxiety disorders.

Undermining Trust:

Anger can erode trust within a family. When family members do not feel emotionally safe or fear unpredictable outbursts, trust in the stability and security of the family unit can be compromised. Trust is essential for maintaining healthy relationships, and anger can undermine this foundation.

Cycles of Violence:

In extreme cases, uncontrolled anger can escalate into physical or emotional abuse. This can create a dangerous cycle of violence within the family, perpetuating a pattern of harm that can have severe and long-lasting consequences.

Impact on Problem Solving:

Anger can hinder effective problem-solving within a family. When individuals are consumed by anger, they may struggle to approach issues calmly and rationally. This can impede the resolution of conflicts and contribute to a cycle of recurring problems.

Social Isolation:

Families experiencing chronic anger may become socially isolated as members withdraw from external relationships due to embarrassment or shame. This isolation can further exacerbate the negative impact of anger on family dynamics.

Financial Consequences:

The consequences of anger may extend beyond emotional and psychological realms to practical aspects of life. For instance, chronic anger may lead to impulsive decision-making, financial irresponsibility, or job loss, affecting the family's overall well-being.

It's important to note that while anger is a natural emotion, learning to manage and express it in constructive ways is crucial for maintaining healthy family relationships. Seeking professional help, such as family therapy or counseling, can be valuable in addressing and resolving issues related to anger within a family.

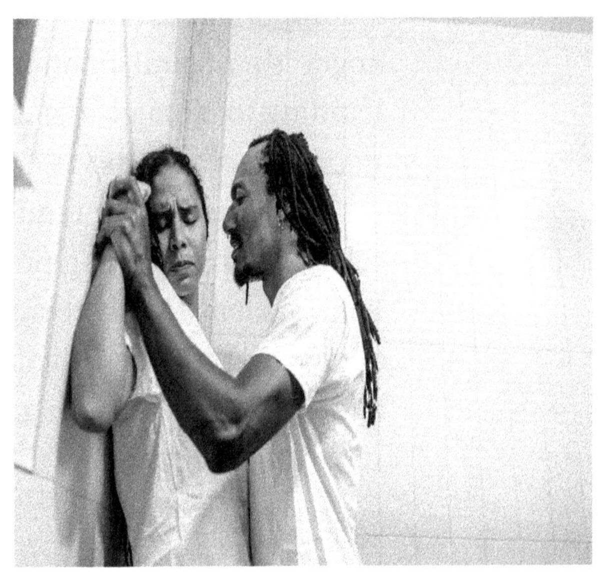

CHAPTER NINE

ROLES OF COMMUNICATION IN ANGER MANAGEMENT

Communication plays a crucial role in anger management, serving as a powerful tool to understand, express, and regulate emotions effectively. Anger is a natural and often healthy emotion, but when it is not managed properly, it can lead to destructive behaviors and strained relationships.

Effective communication can help individuals navigate and diffuse anger by promoting understanding, empathy, and problem-solving. Here's an extensive exploration of the role of communication in anger management:

Self-awareness through Communication:

Communication enables individuals to become more self-aware of their emotions, including anger triggers and the underlying causes. Verbalizing feelings can provide clarity about the source of anger, helping individuals identify whether it stems from frustration, fear, hurt, or other underlying emotions.

Expression of Feelings:

Open and honest communication allows individuals to express their feelings in a constructive manner. Articulating emotions helps in avoiding the buildup of resentment and bitterness, as it prevents emotions from being internalized and turning into explosive anger.

Active Listening:

Effective communication involves active listening, which is crucial in anger management. Listening to others without judgment fosters understanding and empathy. When individuals feel heard and understood, it reduces the intensity of their anger and contributes to a more cooperative and collaborative atmosphere.

Assertive Communication:

Assertive communication involves expressing thoughts, feelings, and needs in a respectful and clear manner, without aggression. Learning assertiveness skills helps individuals communicate their needs and boundaries, reducing the likelihood of feeling ignored or taken advantage of, which can be sources of anger.

Problem-Solving:

Communication is integral to resolving conflicts and addressing the root causes of anger. Engaging in constructive conversations to find solutions promotes a sense of control and empowerment, reducing feelings of helplessness that often contribute to anger.

Emotional Regulation:

Effective communication provides
tools for emotional regulation.
Techniques such as deep breathing,
taking breaks, or using "I"
statements can be communicated
to signal the need for a pause and
self-reflection.
Expressing the need for a timeout
can prevent escalating conflicts
and allow individuals to manage
their emotions before engaging in
a conversation.

Cognitive Restructuring:

Communication plays a role in
cognitive restructuring, which
involves changing negative
thought patterns that contribute to
anger.

Engaging in positive self-talk and challenging irrational thoughts can be communicated both internally and externally, fostering a more positive and balanced perspective.

Building Positive Relationships:

Communication is the foundation to building and maintaining positive relationships. Healthy communication patterns contribute to trust, understanding, and emotional intimacy.
Strong relationships act as a buffer against anger, as individuals feel more supported and connected.

Educational and Therapeutic Interventions:

Communication is a central component of anger management

programs and therapeutic interventions.

Teaching individuals effective communication skills equips them with the tools to express themselves in a way that promotes understanding and minimizes the likelihood of aggressive outbursts. Effective communication is essential for understanding, expressing, and managing anger.

By fostering self-awareness, promoting active listening, and encouraging assertive and constructive communication, individuals can navigate conflicts, build positive relationships, and ultimately develop healthier approaches to anger management.

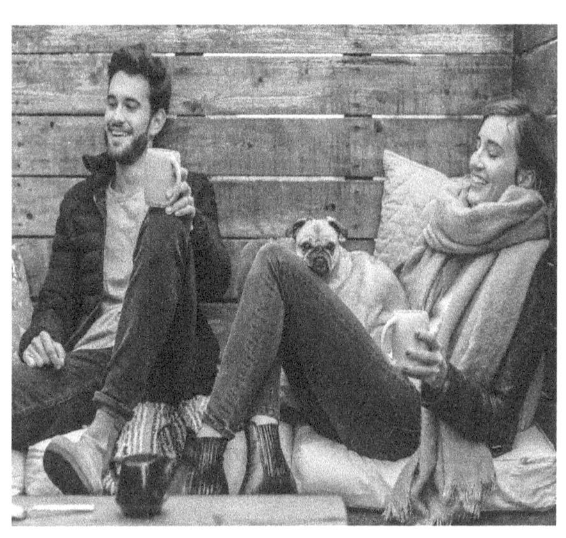

CHAPTER TEN

HOW TO EFFECTIVELY MANAGE ANGER

Yes, anger can be managed. Anger is a normal and natural emotion that everyone experiences, but how it is expressed and dealt with varies from person to person. Effective anger management involves learning to recognize signs of anger, understanding its underlying causes, and developing healthy ways to express and control it.

Recognize Triggers: Identify situations, people, or events that trigger your anger. Awareness of these triggers can help you anticipate and manage your response. Identify the situations, events, or people that tend to trigger your anger. Understanding your triggers is the very first step in managing them perfectly well.

Take a Timeout: If you feel anger rising, take a break before reacting. Step away from the situation, take deep breaths, and give yourself time to cool down.

Express Yourself: Communicate your feelings assertively, but not aggressively. Use "I" statements when expressing how you feel without blaming anyone. For example, say "I feel frustrated when..." instead of "You always make me angry when..."

Practice Relaxation Techniques: Techniques such as deep breathing, meditation, or progressive muscle relaxation can help calm your mind and body, reducing the intensity of anger.

Exercise Regularly: Physical activity is a great way to release built-up tension and reduce stress, which can contribute to anger. Find an exercise routine that you enjoy and can incorporate into your life.

Develop Healthy Outlets: Find positive ways to express and release anger, such as engaging in a hobby, talking to a friend, or journaling. Avoid destructive outlets like substance abuse or aggressive behavior.

Counseling or Therapy: If anger issues persist and significantly impact your life, seeking the help of a mental health professional can provide valuable tools and insights.

Monitor physical cues:

Pay attention to physical signs of anger, such as increased heart rate, muscle tension, or changes in breathing. Being aware of these cues can help you intervene before your anger escalates.

Challenge negative thoughts: Examine and challenge the thoughts that contribute to your anger. Ask yourself if your interpretation of a situation is accurate and whether your reaction is proportionate.

Reframe negative thinking: Replace irrational thoughts with more rational ones. For example, instead of thinking, "This is unfair and I can't stand it," try thinking, "This is challenging, but I can handle it."

Deep breath: Always practice deep, slow breathing in order to

calm your nervous system. Also
try to inhale deeply through your
nose, hold your breath for a few
seconds, and then exhale slowly
through your mouth.

Progressive muscle relaxation:
Tense and then gradually release
each muscle group in your body.
This can help reduce overall
tension and stress.

Take a break: If you feel anger
rising, step away from the
situation. Always give yourself
sometime to cool down and gain
perspective. Physical distance can
prevent impulsive and regrettable
actions or words.

Identify solutions: Instead of
dwelling on the problem, always
more focus on finding solutions.
Collaborate with others to address

the underlying issues causing your anger.

Set realistic expectations: Adjust your expectations to match reality. Unrealistic expectations can lead to frustration and anger.

Seek Support:

Say it out: Sharing your feelings with a trusted friend, family member, colleague or therapist. Sometimes, discussing your anger with someone else can provide a fresh perspective and emotional support.

Adequate sleep: Lack of sleep can contribute to irritability and difficulty managing emotions. Prioritize getting enough rest each night.

Mindfulness practices: Techniques such as meditation, deep breathing, and mindfulness exercises can help you stay present and reduce the intensity of your emotional reactions.

*Mindful awareness:*Pay attention to your thoughts and feelings without judgment. This can help you detach from the immediate emotional response and choose a more measured reaction.

*Professional Help:*After doing the aforementioned, if anger issues persist and significantly impact your life, consider seeking professional help from a therapist or counselor. They will provide additional strategies and support tailored to your specific situation.

*Count to Ten:*Before reacting, count to ten slowly. This simple technique can give you a moment to pause and think before responding impulsively.

Step Away: If possible, physically remove yourself from the situation. Take a short walk, go to a quiet place, or give yourself some space to cool down.

Seek Understanding: Try to understand the source of your anger. Is it related to a specific event, or is it a result of accumulated stress? Understanding the root cause of your anger can help you address the issue effectively.

Set Realistic Expectations:Accept that people, including yourself, are not perfect. Adjust your expectations, and be open to the possibility that things might not always go as planned.

Develop Problem-Solving Skills:
Instead of focusing on blame,
work on finding solutions to the
issues that trigger your anger. This
proactive approach can help
prevent the cycle of aggression.

Managing anger and avoiding
transferring aggression can be
challenging, but it's crucial for
maintaining healthy relationships
and well-being.

Remember that anger is a normal
emotion, but it's crucial to manage
it constructively to maintain
healthy relationships and personal
well-being. Developing these skills
takes time and practice, so be
patient with yourself as you work
towards effective anger
management.

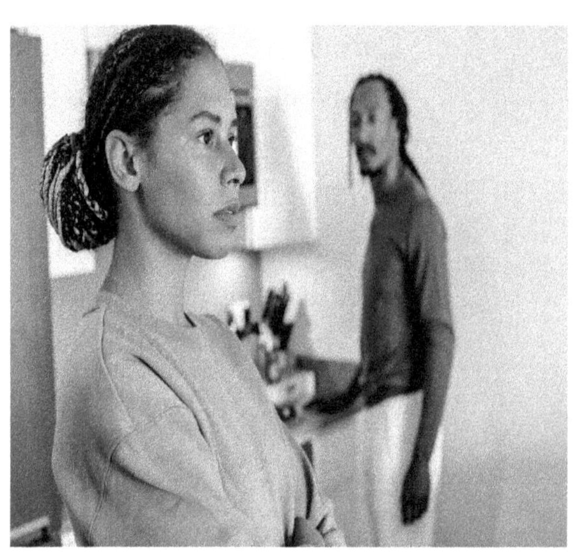

CHAPTER ELEVEN

ANGER MANAGEMENT IN MARRIAGE

Managing anger is crucial in any relationship, and for spouses, it becomes particularly important due to the close and intimate nature of the bond. Uncontrolled anger can lead to conflicts, hurt feelings, and long-lasting damage to the relationship.

Anger is a natural and often unavoidable emotion that can arise in any relationship, including marriage, effective anger management is crucial to maintaining a healthy and thriving marital relationship. Uncontrolled anger can lead to conflict, resentment, and long-term damage to the emotional well-being of both partners. Here, we will explore comprehensive strategies for managing anger in marriage.

Understanding the Root Causes:

It's essential for couples to identify the underlying causes of anger. Often, anger is a manifestation of deeper emotions such as fear, frustration, or hurt. By recognizing and addressing the root causes, couples can work together to find constructive solutions.

Effective Communication:

Communication is key in any relationship, and it becomes even more crucial in the context of anger management. Encourage open and honest communication, but do so in a calm and respectful manner. Using "I" statements instead of "you" statements can help express feelings without blaming the other person.

Active Listening:

Actively listening to your partner is an integral part of effective communication. By giving your full attention and showing empathy, you create an environment where both partners feel heard and understood. This can prevent misunderstandings that often lead to anger.

Developing Emotional Intelligence:

Emotional intelligence involves recognizing, understanding, and managing one's own emotions, as well as being attuned to the emotions of others. Developing emotional intelligence can help individuals regulate their emotions, making it easier to respond to conflict in a more constructive way.

Taking Time-Outs:

When emotions are running high, taking a temporary break can be beneficial. This time-out allows both partners to cool down, collect their thoughts, and approach the issue with a clearer perspective. It's crucial to establish mutually agreed-upon rules for timeouts to prevent them from being misinterpreted as avoidance or abandonment.

If anger issues persist and become a recurring problem, seeking the assistance of a marriage counselor or therapist can be invaluable. A neutral third party can provide guidance, teach effective coping mechanisms, and help both partners navigate through challenging emotions.

Cultivating Empathy:

Empathy includes understanding and sharing in the feelings of another. Cultivating empathy in a marriage can create a stronger emotional connection. When partners can put themselves in each other's shoes, it fosters understanding and diminishes the likelihood of explosive reactions to triggers.

Constructive Problem-Solving:

Instead of focusing on blame, work together to find solutions to the issues causing anger. Develop problem-solving skills that allow both partners to express their needs and work towards common goals. This collaborative approach reinforces the idea that the couple is a team, facing challenges together.

Healthy Outlets for Stress:

Encouraging each other to engage in activities that help manage stress can contribute to a more balanced emotional state. This might include exercise, hobbies, or relaxation techniques that provide an outlet for negative emotions before they escalate.

Establishing Boundaries:

Clearly defined boundaries can prevent situations that trigger anger. Discuss and agree upon acceptable behavior and communication guidelines. Having a shared understanding of each other's limits helps create a more respectful and considerate relationship.

Recognize Triggers:

Be aware of personal triggers that lead to anger. Understanding what sets off your anger can help you and your spouse navigate potential conflicts.

Seek Solutions, Not Blame:

Focus more on finding solutions to problems rather than placing blame on others. A collaborative approach fosters a sense of teamwork in the relationship.

Practice Relaxation Techniques:

Incorporate relaxation techniques such as deep breathing, meditation, or mindfulness to manage stress and prevent anger from escalating.

Apologize and Forgive:

Apologize sincerely when you are in the wrong, and forgive your partner when they make mistakes. Holding onto grudges can fuel ongoing anger.

Develop a Sense of Humor:

Humor can be a powerful tool in diffusing tension. Finding moments of levity can break the cycle of anger and bring a lighter perspective to the situation.

Work on Self-Awareness:

Reflect on your own emotional responses and patterns. Increased self-awareness can lead to better self-regulation and understanding of your triggers.

Celebrate Positives:

Focus on positive aspects of the relationship. Expressing gratitude and appreciation can create a more positive atmosphere, reducing the likelihood of anger.

Anger management in marriage is a dynamic process that requires ongoing effort and commitment from both partners. By fostering effective communication, emotional intelligence, and a collaborative approach to problem-solving, couples can navigate conflicts in a way that strengthens their connection rather than erodes it. Seeking professional help when needed is a sign of strength and a proactive step towards building a resilient and fulfilling marital relationship. Remember, managing anger is an ongoing process that requires commitment and effort from both partners. By adopting these strategies, spouses can build a healthier and more resilient relationship.

CHAPTER TWELVE

PARENT-KID ANGER MANAGEMENT

Anger is a natural emotion that everyone experiences, including parents and children. However, managing anger effectively is crucial for maintaining healthy relationships within the family.

Uncontrolled anger can lead to strained parent-child relationships, emotional distress, and even long-term psychological effects on children. Here's an extensive exploration of anger management for both parents and kids:

Anger Management for Parents:

1. Recognize Triggers:
Parents should identify specific situations or behaviors that trigger their anger. Understanding these triggers can help in developing strategies to avoid or cope with them.

2. Pause and Reflect:
Before reacting in anger, parents should take a moment to pause and reflect on their emotions. This brief moment of reflection can prevent impulsive and regrettable actions.

3. Communication Skills:
Effective communication is key. Parents should express their feelings calmly and assertively, using "I" statements to avoid

sounding accusatory as this fosters an open and understanding atmosphere.

4. Stress Management:
High stress levels can contribute to heightened anger. Parents should prioritize self-care, incorporating stress-reducing activities such as exercise, meditation, or hobbies into their routine.

5. Set Realistic Expectations:
Unrealistic expectations of children's behavior can lead to frustration. Parents should establish age-appropriate expectations and recognize that children are still learning and developing.

6. Seek Support:
It's essential for parents to have a support system. Whether it's through friends, family, or

counseling, having someone to talk to can provide perspective and guidance.

7. Model Healthy Behavior: Parents serve as role models for their children. Demonstrating healthy anger management techniques teaches kids how to handle their emotions constructively.

8. Apologize and Repair: Everyone makes mistakes. When parents do lose their temper, it's crucial to apologize and discuss the situation afterward. This teaches children the importance of taking responsibility for one's actions.

ANGER MANAGEMENT FOR KIDS:

1. Identify Feelings:
Children need to learn to recognize and label their emotions, including anger. This self-awareness is the first step in managing their feelings.

2. Breathing Exercises:
Teaching children simple breathing exercises can help them calm down when they feel angry. Deep breaths can slow heart rate and bring a sense of control.

3. Use "I" Statements:
Always encourage a child or children to express their feelings

using "I" statements. For example,
saying "I feel upset when..." is
more constructive than blaming
others.

4. Problem-Solving Skills:
Help children develop
problem-solving skills to address
the root causes of their anger. This
empowers them to find
constructive solutions rather than
reacting impulsively.

5. Time-Outs and Safe Spaces:
Establishing a designated space or
time-out method allows children to
step away and cool down when
emotions run high.

6. Teach Coping Strategies:
Encourage the use of positive
coping mechanisms like drawing,
journaling, or engaging in physical
activities as alternatives to
expressing anger.

7. Reward Positive Behavior:
Positive reinforcement can be a
powerful tool. Acknowledge and
reward children when they handle
their anger appropriately,
reinforcing those positive
behaviors.

8. Family Meetings:
Regular family meetings does
provide a platform for open
communication. Encourage
children to express their feelings
and concerns in a safe
environment.

However, effective anger
management for parents and
children involves self-awareness,
communication, and the
development of coping strategies.
By fostering a supportive and
understanding family environment,
both parents and children can learn

to navigate and express their
emotions in a healthy and
constructive manner.

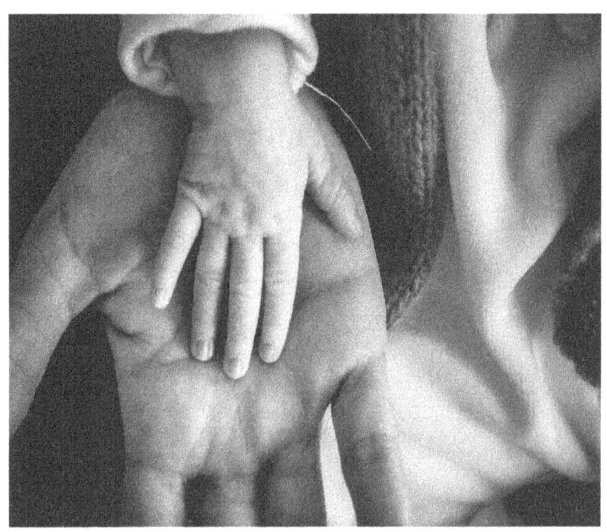

CHAPTER THIRTEEN

MAINTAINING HEALTHY RELATIONSHIP VOID OF CONFLICT

Building and maintaining healthy relationships void of conflict requires intentional effort, effective communication, and a commitment to understanding and respecting each other. Here are some good tips that can help you achieve that:
Building Healthy Relationships:

Communication:

Active Listening: Make an effort to understand the other person's perspective. Listen without interrupting and show empathy.

Express Yourself: Clearly communicate your thoughts, feelings, and needs. Be honest and open.

Respect:

Boundaries: Respect personal boundaries and be mindful of each other's space, both physical and emotional.

Differences: Acknowledge and appreciate the differences between you and the other person.

Empathy:

Put Yourself in Their Shoes: Try to understand the other person's feelings and experiences. This can foster a deeper connection.

Trust:

Reliability: Be consistent and reliable in your actions. Trust is built over time through consistency and follow-through.

Transparency: Be open and honest. Avoid keeping secrets or hiding information.

Positivity:

Focus on the Positive: Acknowledge and appreciate the positive aspects of the relationship. Express gratitude for each other.

Quality Time:

Invest Time Together: Spend quality time with each other to strengthen your connection. This can involve shared activities and meaningful conversations.

Compromise:

Flexibility: Be willing to compromise when necessary. Sometimes finding common ground is essential for long-term harmony.

Resolving and Managing Conflict:

Timely Discussions: Address issues as they arise rather than letting them fester.

Always use "I" Statements:
Always express your feelings and concerns using "I" statements to avoid blaming someone.

Conflict Resolution Skills:

Problem Solving: Always focus on finding solutions rather than dwelling on the problem(s).
Seek Common Grounds: Always find areas of agreement and build on them.

Understanding:

Perspective-Taking: Try to understand the other person's point of view, even if you disagree. This can defuse tension.

Stay Calm:

Emotional Regulation: Avoid escalating conflicts by managing your emotions. Always take a break if need be to cool off before continuing the discussion.

Forgiveness:

Let Go: Always forgive and move forward. Holding onto grudges may erode the foundation of your relationship.

Learn and Grow:

Reflect: After conflicts, reflect on what happened and how you can both learn and grow from the experience.

Professional Help:

Therapy: If conflicts persist, consider seeking the help of a professional therapist or counselor to facilitate communication.

Remember, no relationship is perfect, and occasional conflicts are normal. The key is to address them constructively and work together to build a stronger, healthier connection.

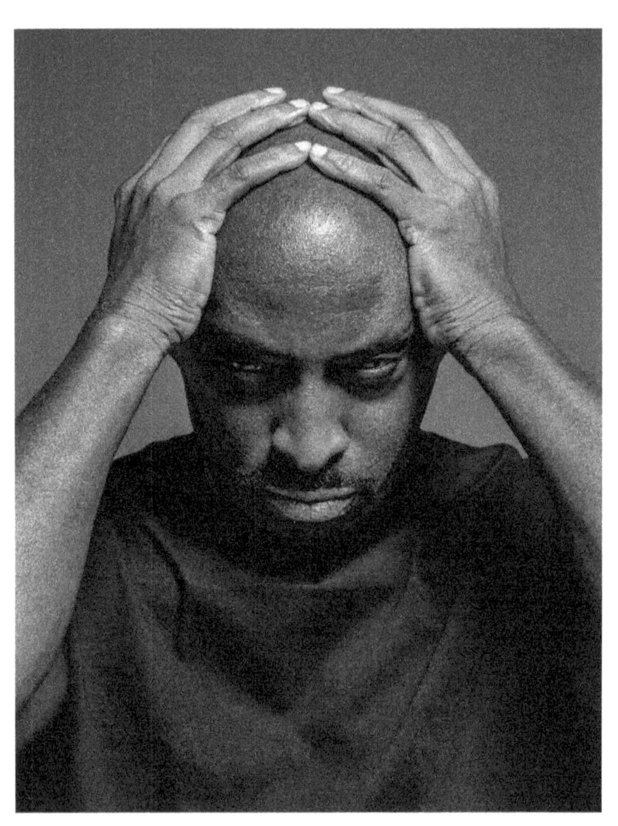

CHAPTER FOURTEEN

EMBRACE SELF-LOVE AMID ANGER

Learning to love yourself and forgiving others are interconnected processes that involve self-awareness, compassion, and a willingness to let go of negative emotions.

In the intricate dance of human emotions, anger often emerges as a formidable force, capable of influencing our thoughts, actions, and relationships.

However, within the realm of self-love lies a transformative power—an antidote that not only

soothes the flames of anger but also fosters a deeper understanding of ourselves. This journey towards self-love in the context of anger is a profound exploration of compassion, forgiveness, and acceptance.
Practice Self-Compassion:
Learn to treat yourself with the same kindness and understanding that you would offer to friends, colleagues, neighbors and family.

Acknowledge your own imperfections and mistakes without harsh self-judgment.

Reflect on Your Own Growth:

Recognize your personal development and the lessons you've learned from your experiences.
Celebrate the positive changes you've made in your life.

Understand the Power of
Forgiveness:

Realize that forgiveness is not
about condoning the other person's
actions but about freeing yourself
from the burden of resentment.
Understand that holding onto
anger and resentment can have a
negative impact on your mental
and emotional well-being.

Cultivate Empathy:

Always try to understand the
perspective of the person(s) you
need to forgive as empathy can
foster compassion and make it
easier to let go of negative
feelings.
Remember that everyone makes
mistakes, and we are all human.

Set Boundaries:

In all, establish healthy boundaries
to protect yourself and people
around you from further harm.
This doesn't mean holding onto
resentment but ensuring that you're
not exposed to repeated negative
behavior.

Practice Mindfulness:

Engage in mindfulness and
meditation practices to stay present
and focused on the current
moment.
Mindfulness can help you observe
your thoughts and emotions
without being overwhelmed by
them.

Seek Support:

Talk to friends, family, or a mental
health professional about your

feelings and the process of
forgiveness.
Sharing your thoughts and
emotions with others can provide
valuable insights and support.

Let Go of Perfectionism:

Accept that everyone, including
yourself and others, is imperfect.
Avoid holding unrealistic
expectations for yourself and those
around you.

Forgive Yourself:

Before forgiving others, learn to
forgive yourself for any mistakes
or perceived shortcomings.
Self-forgiveness is an essential part
of cultivating a compassionate and
loving relationship with yourself.
Focus on the Present and Future:

Redirect your energy toward the present moment and future rather than dwelling on past grievances. Set goals and aspirations that align with your values and contribute to your personal growth.

The synergy between self-love and anger is a dynamic process of self-discovery and growth. By understanding the roots of anger, practicing self-reflection, and embracing forgiveness, individuals can forge a path toward a more compassionate and resilient self. In the tapestry of human emotions, self-love is the thread that weaves together understanding, acceptance, and the capacity to navigate the complex landscape of anger with grace and empathy.

CHAPTER FIFTEEN

TIPS TO HANDLE DIFFICULT SITUATIONS

Handling difficult situations requires a combination of emotional intelligence, problem-solving skills, and effective communication. These tips may be helpful:

Stay Calm:

Try to remain calm and composed. Take a few deep breaths to manage your stress and emotions.
Keeping a level head allows you to think more clearly and make better decisions.

Understand the Situation:

Take the time to fully understand the situation before reacting. Gather as much information as possible.
Consider the perspectives of others involved to gain a comprehensive understanding.

Focus on Solutions:

Instead of dwelling on the problems, adjust your focus to finding good solutions.
Break down the problem into smaller or more manageable parts.

Communicate Effectively:

Clearly express your thoughts and concerns. Always use "I" statements to avoid sounding accusatory when airing your view.

Always listen actively to others
and try to understand their
perspectives too.

Empathy:

Put yourself in another's situation
to understand their feelings and
motivations.
Demonstrating empathy can help
build rapport and foster a more
cooperative atmosphere.

Set Boundaries:

Clearly define your boundaries and
assert them when necessary.
Establishing healthy boundaries is
important for maintaining your
well-being.

Learn from the Experience:

Treat difficult situations as
learning opportunities. Consider

what you can take away from the
experience to improve in the
future.
Reflect on your actions and
identify areas that can help your
personal growth.

Seek Support:

Don't hesitate to seek help from
friends, family and colleagues.
Discussing the situation with
others can provide valuable
perspectives and emotional
support.

Take Breaks:

If the situation becomes
overwhelming, take breaks to give
yourself time to regroup and
recharge.
Stepping away briefly can help
you gain a fresh perspective.

Problem-Solving Skills:

Develop and enhance your problem-solving skills. Always break down complex problems into smaller and more manageable steps.
Consider alternative solutions and weigh their pros and cons.

Adaptability:

Be flexible and open to adapting your approach as the situation evolves.
Rigidity can exacerbate difficult situations, so be willing to consider different perspectives and solutions.

Maintain a Positive Mindset:

Focus on positive aspects, even in challenging situations. A positive mindset can help you approach problems with optimism and resilience.

Every difficult situation is unique, and the effectiveness of these tips may vary. It's essential to tailor your approach based on the specific circumstances you're facing.

CHAPTER SIXTEEN

LET GO GRUDGES

Letting go of grudges can be a challenging but important step for your own emotional well-being. Holding onto resentment and anger can negatively impact your mental and physical health. Here are some steps you can take to let go of grudges:

Acknowledge Your Feelings:

Recognize and accept the emotions you're experiencing. It is very okay to feel angry, hurt, or upset.

Understand the Impact on You:

Consider the toll that holding onto a grudge is taking on your own well-being. Understand that forgiveness is more about your peace of mind than excusing the other person's behavior.

Empathize with the Other Person:

Always try to see some situations from the other person's perspective. This doesn't mean condoning their actions, but understanding their motivations or circumstances can help you empathize.

Detach Yourself from the
Situation:

Understand that holding onto a grudge ties you to the negative emotions associated with the past. Choose to detach yourself from the situation and focus on the present and future.

Practice Self-Compassion:

Be kind to yourself. Understand that forgiveness is a process, and it's okay if it takes time. Don't be too hard on yourself for having negative emotions.

Express Your Feelings:

Always talk about your feelings with a trusted friend, colleague, family member, or therapist. Expressing your emotions can be cathartic and can help you gain perspective.

If it feels appropriate and safe, consider communicating with the person involved. This doesn't necessarily mean reconciling, but it can help you express your feelings and possibly gain closure.

Focus on the Present:
Redirect your energy towards positive aspects of your life by engaging in activities that bring you joy, and cultivate a positive mindset.

Mindfulness techniques and meditation can help you stay present and let go of negative thoughts associated with the grudge.

If letting go of a grudge is particularly challenging, consider seeking the help of a therapist or counselor. They can provide guidance and support in navigating through your emotions.

Forgiveness doesn't mean condoning the actions of the other person; it means releasing the hold those actions have on your own life. It's a process that takes time and effort, but it can lead to greater emotional freedom and well-being.
Top of Form

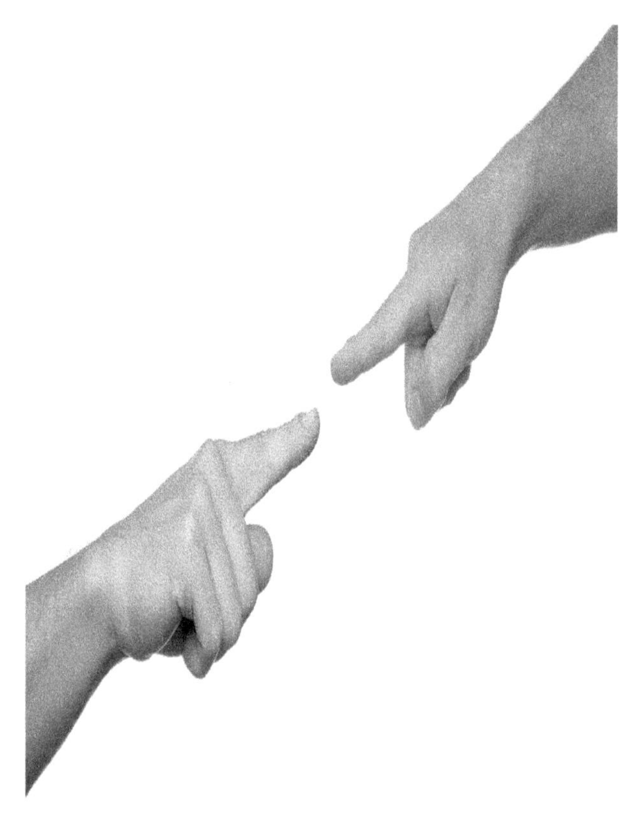

CHAPTER SEVENTEEN

ANGER AND PRODUCTIVITY

Channeling anger into something productive requires a conscious and intentional effort to transform negative emotions into positive actions. Unchecked anger can be destructive both to yourself and others, but when harnessed properly, it can serve as a powerful motivator for positive change. Here are some strategies to help you channel anger into something productive:

1. Acknowledge and Accept Your Anger:
Recognize that anger is a natural emotion, and it's okay to feel it.

Avoid suppressing or denying your anger, as this can lead to more significant issues later.

2. Take a Step Back:
Before you react impulsively, please do take a moment to step back and gain some perspectives. Give yourself time to cool down and think more rationally about the situation.

3. Understand the Source:
Identify the root cause of your anger. Is it a specific event, a pattern of behavior, or an unresolved issue? Understanding the source helps you address the underlying problem.

4. Practice Mindfulness and Deep Breathing:
Engage in mindfulness techniques to stay present in the moment. Deep breathing exercises can help

calm your nervous system and provide a buffer between your emotions and your actions.

5. Express Yourself Constructively:
Communicate your feelings in a calm and assertive manner. Always use "I" statements to express how the situation is affecting you instead of placing blame. This can facilitate a more productive conversation.

6. Seek Solutions:
Rather than dwelling on the negative aspects of a situation, focus more on finding solutions. Channel your energy into problem-solving rather than ruminating on the anger itself.

7. Physical Activity:
Engage in physical activities to release built-up tension. Exercise

is an excellent way to channel anger into something positive and healthy. It can also promote the release of endorphins, which are natural mood elevators.

8. Creative Outlets:
Channel your anger into creative pursuits such as writing, art, music, or any other form of self-expression. This can serve as a cathartic release and help you transform negative energy into something positive.

9. Set Goals:
Use your anger as fuel to set and achieve meaningful goals. Channeling your energy into productive endeavors can give you a sense of accomplishment and purpose.

10. Educate Yourself:

If your anger is related to a specific issue, invest time in educating yourself about it. This knowledge can empower you to advocate for positive change and make a meaningful impact.

Practice Empathy:

Always try to understand the perspectives of others involved in the situation no matter what happened. Empathy can help diffuse anger and open the door to more constructive communication.

Professional Help:

If anger becomes a persistent and overwhelming issue, consider seeking professional help. Therapy or counseling can provide you with tools to manage anger and explore its underlying causes.

Learn from the Experience:

Use moments of anger as opportunities for personal growth. Reflect on your reactions and identify ways to handle similar situations more effectively in the future.

The goal is not to eliminate anger entirely but to channel it into actions that promote positive change and personal development. By adopting these strategies, you can transform anger from a potentially harmful force into a catalyst for growth and improvement.

CHAPTER EIGHTEEN

ANGER Q&A

Certainly, it's important to approach the topic of anger with sensitivity. When creating an anger questionnaire, consider the purpose and audience. Here's a general anger questionnaire that you can use or modify based on your specific needs:

Anger Questionnaire

Section 1: Personal Information

1.1. Name: [**Optional**]
1.2. Age:
1.3. Gender:
1.4. Occupation:

1.5. Relationship Status:

Section 2: Anger Triggers

2.1. What situations or events typically trigger your anger?
2.2. Do you notice any patterns in the triggers for your anger? (e.g., specific people, environments, or circumstances)
2.3. On a scale of 1 to 10, how intense is your anger during these triggers? (1 = mild irritation, 10 = extreme rage)

Section 3: Anger Expression

3.1. How do you typically express your anger? (e.g., yelling, silent treatment, physical actions)
3.2. Do you feel in control of your anger when expressing it, or do you feel it takes over?

3.3. Have you ever regretted how you expressed your anger? If so, please provide an example.

Section 4: Coping Mechanisms

4.1. What strategies do you currently use to cope with anger?
4.2. How effective do you find these strategies in managing your anger? (e.g., very effective, somewhat effective, not effective at all)
4.3. Are there any coping mechanisms you would like to try or improve upon?

Section 5: Impact on Relationships

5.1. How does your anger impact your relationships with family, friends, or colleagues?

5.2. Have you received feedback from others about your anger, and if so, how did you react to it?
5.3. Do you think your anger has led to any strained relationships? If yes, how would you like to address or improve these relationships?

Section 6: Seeking Support

6.1. Have you ever sought professional help or counseling for issues related to anger?
6.2. If not, what factors have influenced your decision not to seek help?
6.3. Would you be open to seeking support or counseling for managing anger in the future?

Section 7: Reflection and Goal Setting

7.1. What are your personal goals for managing anger more effectively?

7.2. How do you envision a positive change in your life if you were able to manage your anger more constructively?

7.3. Is there anything else you would like to share about your experiences with anger?

ANGER QUESTIONNAIRE FOR MEN

Instructions: Please answer the following questions honestly by indicating the most appropriate response for each statement.

On a scale of 1 to 10, with 1 being not at all and 10 being extremely, how would you rate your overall level of anger in daily life?

1

2

3

4

5

6

7

8

9

10

How do you typically express your anger? Please check all that apply.

Verbal outbursts

Physical aggression

Silent treatment

Passive-aggressive behavior

Sarcasm

Withdrawal

Other (please specify):

____

What are the most common triggers for your anger? Check all that apply.

Work-related stress
Relationship issues
Financial concerns
Health problems
Traffic or commuting
Family matters
Other (please specify):

____

How do you feel immediately after
expressing anger?
Relieved
Guilty
Regretful
Empowered
Resentful
Other (please specify):

____

How often do you find yourself
thinking about past situations that
made you angry?
Rarely
Occasionally
Frequently
Almost constantly

Do you believe that your anger has negatively impacted your relationships?

Yes

No

Unsure

What strategies do you currently use to manage your anger? Check all that apply.

Taking deep breaths

Counting to ten

Physical exercise

Talking to someone about it

Taking a break or timeout

Seeking professional help

Other (please specify):

____

How willing are you to seek help or attend anger management programs if you believe it would be beneficial?

Very willing

Somewhat willing

Neutral

Somewhat unwilling

Very unwilling

In your opinion, how does societal expectations of masculinity contribute to how men express or suppress their anger?

Strongly agree

Agree

Neutral

Disagree

Strongly disagree

Is there anything else you would like to share about your experience with anger or how you handle it?

ANGER QUESTIONNAIRE FOR WOMEN

Note: Participants can respond on a scale (e.g., 1 to 5), where 1 is "strongly disagree" and 5 is "strongly agree," or you can use a Likert scale.

Demographic Information:

Age:
Occupation:
Marital Status:

Educational Background:

General Anger Expression:
On a scale from 1 to 5, how often do you feel angry?

How do you generally express your anger? (e.g., verbal expression, physical activity, withdrawal)

What situations or events tend to trigger your anger?
How well do you think you understand the root causes of your anger?

Do you experience physical symptoms when you're angry? (e.g., increased heart rate, tension headaches)
How would you describe the intensity of your physical reactions to anger?

Coping Mechanisms:

What strategies do you use to cope with anger? (e.g., deep breathing, talking to someone, taking a break)
How effective do you find these strategies in managing your anger?

Communication Style:

How would you describe your communication style when you're angry? (e.g., assertive, passive, aggressive)
Do you feel that your communication style is influenced by societal expectations for women?

Impact on Relationships:

In your experience, how has anger affected your relationships, both personally and professionally?

How do you believe others
perceive your expressions of
anger?

Cultural and Gender Influences:

To what extent do you feel societal
expectations and cultural norms
impact how you express or
suppress your anger as a woman?

Seeking Support:

How comfortable are you seeking
support or discussing your anger
with others?
Have you ever sought professional
help or counseling to address
issues related to anger?

Self-Reflection:

How would you rate your level of self-awareness regarding your anger?

What steps, if any, do you take to reflect on and understand your emotions, including anger?

Consider the specific context in which you plan to use this questionnaire and make any necessary adjustments. Additionally, ensure that participants are aware of the purpose and confidentiality of the assessment.

CHAPTER NINETEEN

CONCLUSION

Effective anger management for men is an essential aspect of promoting mental and emotional well-being, fostering healthy relationships, and contributing to a more harmonious society. Recognizing that anger is a natural emotion, the emphasis lies in developing constructive strategies to channel and express this emotion in a way that is both assertive and respectful.

The journey towards effective anger management involves self-awareness, where individuals gain insight into their triggers, warning signs, and the root causes of their anger. Equally important is the cultivation of emotional intelligence, empowering men to understand and navigate their emotions with greater finesse. Education and awareness-raising play crucial roles, dismantling societal stereotypes that may discourage men from seeking help or expressing vulnerability. Furthermore, the implementation of practical techniques, such as mindfulness, deep-breathing exercises, and cognitive restructuring, equips men with the tools needed to regulate their emotional responses.

Communication skills also play a pivotal role, enabling men to express themselves assertively without resorting to aggression, and fostering healthier interactions with others.
Engaging in therapy or support groups provides a structured and

professional environment for men to explore the underlying issues contributing to their anger, fostering personal growth and resilience.

Additionally, creating a culture that encourages open dialogue around emotions and mental health reduces the stigma associated with seeking help.

Ultimately, the goal of anger management for men is not to eliminate anger but to transform it into a constructive force. By embracing a holistic approach that combines self-awareness, emotional intelligence, practical techniques, and support systems, men can develop a healthier relationship with their anger. This, in turn, promotes positive mental health outcomes, strengthens interpersonal connections, and

contributes to the creation of a
more empathetic and
understanding society.

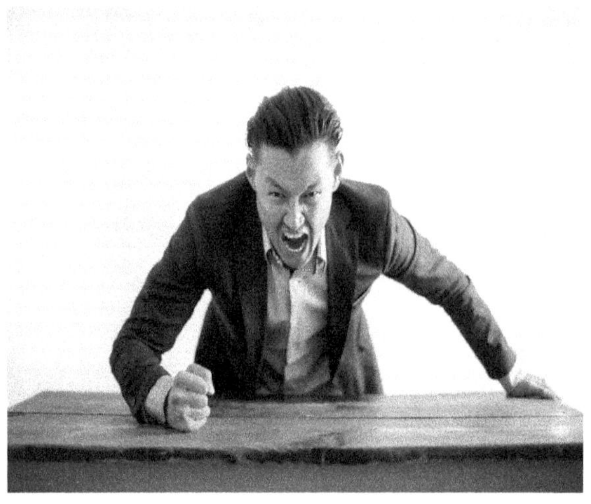

www.ingramcontent.com/pod-product-compliance
Lightning Source LLC
Chambersburg PA
CBHW071603270726
48661CB00018B/1074